What readers are saying about IN 30 MINUTES® guides:

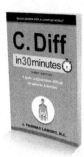

C. Diff In 30 Minutes

"This book is very informational about all things C. diff. It reiterated what my son's doctors have been saying and gave me comfort that they know the proper way to treat C. diff."

"I am glad there was a book that could answer my questions about C. diff, and to know other people were in the same boat as me."

Genealogy Basics In 30 Minutes

"This basic genealogy book is a fast, informative read that will get you on your way if you are ready to begin your genealogy journey or are looking for tips to push past a problem area."

"The personal one-on-one feel and the obvious dedication it took to boil down a lot of research into such a small book and still make it readable are the two reasons I give this book such a high rating. Recommended."

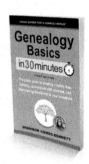

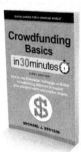

Crowdfunding Basics In 30 Minutes

"Very understandable and absorbing. A must-read for any entrepreneur."

"On the verge of launching a crowdfunding campaign myself, this book has made me re-think my plans and my strategy. Take a step back and get the advice of someone who's been there."

Twitter In 30 Minutes

"A perfect introduction to Twitter. Quick and easy read with lots of photos. I finally understand the # symbol!"

"Clarified any issues and concerns I had and listed some excellent precautions."

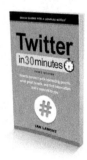

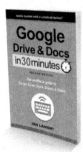

Google Drive & Docs In 30 Minutes

"I bought your Google Docs guide myself (my new company uses it) and it was really handy. I loved it."

"I have been impressed by the writing style and how easy it was to get very familiar and start leveraging Google Docs. I can't wait for more titles. Nice job!"

Learn more about IN 30 MINUTES® guides at in30minutes.com

Acid Reflux & Heartburn

In 30 Minutes

A guide to acid reflux, heartburn, and GERD for patients and families

FIRST EDITION

By J. Thomas Lamont, M.D.

IN 30 MINUTES® Guides

Published by i30 Media Corporation
Newton, Massachusetts

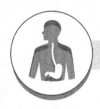

Contents

Contents

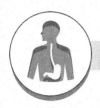

Foreword

Welcome to *Acid Reflux & Heartburn In 30 Minutes*. If you or a family member are among the millions of people suffering from heartburn or a more serious condition called acid reflux or gastroesophageal reflux disease (GERD), you are dealing with discomfort that impacts many areas of life, from eating to sleeping.

This guide is intended to help answer basic questions about heartburn and GERD, and to reassure patients and family members. While some patients experience the symptoms of heartburn and GERD on a daily basis and despair that they will ever recover, there are in fact a range of treatment options that can offer relief. Of course, any treatment of heartburn and GERD must be made after discussions with your doctor.

The author of *Acid Reflux & Heartburn In 30 Minutes* is Gastroenterologist and Harvard Medical School Professor, Dr. J. Thomas Lamont. Over the past three decades, Dr. Lamont has treated thousands of patients suffering from heartburn and GERD. Using plain English, he will explain the basics of heartburn and acid reflux, ranging from causes to treatments. He will also explore more specific topics, such as:

➤ How your stomach works

➤ How reflux occurs

➤ Heartburn symptoms

➤ Diagnosing acid reflux

➤ Trigger foods

➤ Lifestyle changes for reflux control

➤ Medications, from antacids to acid blockers

➤ Surgical procedures to treat acid reflux

The author also describes four cases involving heartburn and GERD. Through the stories of an obese patient, a pregnant woman and new mother, a 64-year-old suffering from severe acid reflux, and a college student, you'll learn how heartburn and GERD impact the lives of ordinary people, the types of treatment that are available, and what the road to recovery looks like.

Acid Reflux & Heartburn In 30 Minutes also includes a glossary of terms and medications, located at the back of the guide and online at *heartburn. in30minutes.com*. The companion website contains additional resources, such as an online glossary, videos, and other information of use to patients suffering from heartburn and GERD.

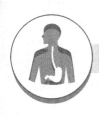

Stomach acid: the good, the bad, and the ugly

Every time you eat, your stomach produces a very powerful acid solution called *gastric juice* that contains the following elements:

➤ **Stomach acid**, a corrosive substance that is secreted by your stomach. Stomach acid is also known as hydrochloric acid.

➤ **Digestive enzymes** that help your body break down and digest your food.

➤ **Bile**, a substance that breaks down fat in your diet.

Stomach acid kills bacteria, viruses, and other harmful germs in our water and food. That's the good news.

Here's the bad news: stomach acid is so strong that it can sometimes burn the lining of the stomach and esophagus, leading to an uncomfortable condition called acid indigestion heartburn, or *agida*. Too much acid in your stomach can even burn a hole or ulcer in the stomach lining.

Heartburn is a symptom of *acid reflux*, in which stomach acid travels upward into the esophagus, where it irritates the lining and causes a burning sensation behind the breast bone. Patients may also experience excessive burping and nausea. The medical name for this condition is gastroesophageal reflux disease, or GERD. Patients usually refer to their problem as heartburn or acid reflux.

Scope of the heartburn problem

About 50 to 60 million Americans report occasional or on-again, off-again heartburn every week or so. Ten to 15 million individuals experience acid reflux on a daily basis. That's why antacid tablets like Tums and Rolaids are sold everywhere, including airports, food markets, and highway rest stops.

People of all ages can get acid reflux, from infants to seniors. However, there are variations among age groups and global populations. In the United States, women are more likely to be diagnosed with reflux-related symptoms, as shown in Figure 1.

Figure 1: Primary or secondary reflux-related hospital diagnoses

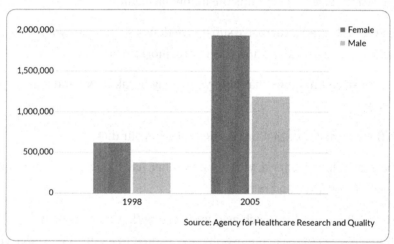

Pregnant women are especially prone to heartburn, particularly in the last trimester when the fetus grows to full size and pushes up on the stomach, forcing acid into the esophagus. In Chapter 1, we'll learn about Evie, a young woman who experienced heartburn when pregnant with her first child.

Some patients notice the onset of heartburn after putting on weight. Others say their heartburn may improve after they lose excess weight. Obesity increases the risk for heartburn. The recent epidemic of weight gain and obesity in industrialized societies has led to a parallel increase in heartburn in all age groups (see Figure 2). Similar to pregnancy, extra fat in the belly pushes upwards on the stomach and forces acid up into the esophagus.

Figure 2: Global prevalence of heartburn and/or acid reflux

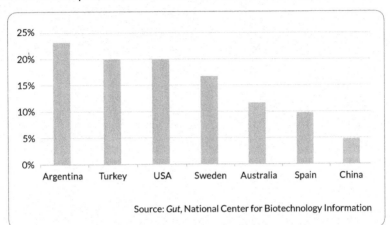

Source: *Gut*, National Center for Biotechnology Information

Certain eating and drinking habits may also aggravate reflux. Many patients notice heartburn or chest discomfort after a rich or spicy meal, such as spaghetti and meatballs in a heavy tomato sauce, washed down with a glass or two of red wine, then followed by a piece of chocolate cake and a cup of coffee. Heavy meals like this are typically consumed in the evening, and are often followed by bad heartburn later that night. Another heartburn scenario is a big breakfast of bacon, eggs, fried potatoes, orange juice, and coffee. Taking a nap after a Sunday brunch like this can bring on a bad attack of heartburn.

While these foods often trigger heartburn and GERD, they are not the root cause. To understand why so many people experience the symptoms, it's necessary to understand how your stomach processes food. We'll explore this topic in Chapter 2. In Chapter 3, I will describe how doctors diagnose heartburn and acid reflux. Then, we'll take a look at treatments in chapters 4 and 5.

But first, let's explore several case studies based on actual patients I have seen and treated. Their situations may shed some light on your experience—and demonstrate that even the most serious cases can be successfully treated.

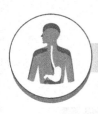
The many faces of acid reflux

What follows are four case histories of people who experienced acid reflux. Their names, identities, and other details have been changed to protect their privacy, and the photos are not of real patients.

You, a friend or a family member may have experiences similar to those of Joe, Evie, Dana, and Jeremy. While these patients are quite different, they share a few things in common—all had severe heartburn that required medical intervention and intensive therapy to block acid production in the stomach. Even though GERD impacted their lives and caused worry for family members, the good news is that all eventually recovered and have returned to their original health status.

Note that certain tests and treatments require professional evaluation and medicines available only by prescription, so the information below is not a do-it-yourself guide. It is provided to help you understand what your doctor is recommending and why.

Joe Leone's case history: "Doc, I can't sleep anymore with this heartburn."

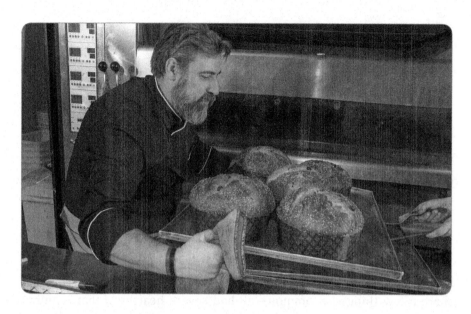

Joe Leone was referred to me because he was experiencing heartburn that just wouldn't go away. This symptom started just after he turned 40. For the next few years, it got progressively worse, to the point that it was seriously impacting his quality of life.

In our initial consultation, he related that he was fine until age 40, then everything started going downhill. But as I asked questions about his medical history, it became apparent that other issues had started earlier. His weight had begun creeping up in his mid-30s, finally reaching 250 pounds in his late 30s. With the extra weight, his blood pressure went up, and he noted that going up stairs made him short of breath.

In fact, Joe worked as a chef in his family's Italian restaurant. It was a job he loved. But his work involved constant exposure to food, not to mention relentless stress from running a business. This combination led to overeating, no time for exercise, and eventually significant obesity.

His family doctor diagnosed Joe with *metabolic syndrome,* a condition associated with central obesity (fat in the belly, but not in the limbs), fat deposits in the liver, high blood pressure, and elevated blood sugar (pre-diabetes). After he started to complain of heartburn, his family doctor prescribed an acid blocker, a medication designed to reduce the production of stomach acid.

Initially the acid reflux got better, and for a time he was able to stop the medicine. But as his weight crept up and his waistline expanded, the heartburn returned worse than before. To control it, Joe was prescribed an acid blocker twice per day. He also kept a bottle of antacid tablets (Tums) on his nightstand to take when a burning discomfort in his chest woke him. Eventually, he was referred to me.

> **What the research says:** In survey data published in the Journal of the American Board of Family Medicine, 63% of respondents who reported more heartburn at night said they had difficulty sleeping, and 40% reported that it impacted daily functioning the following day. (Source: *Journal of the American Board of Family Medicine*, 2005.)

When I took his history, I learned that Joe didn't like the idea of taking medication on a regular basis. His referring doctor also mentioned that Joe's blood pressure was very difficult to control, and that he suspected that Joe was not taking his blood pressure pills on a regular basis.

When I questioned Joe about taking his heartburn medications, Joe said that his approach was to take these medications only when his heartburn was especially bothersome.

"Some days I don't have as much heartburn," he said. "So I figure I can lay off the meds."

I explained to Joe that acid blocking medication needs to be taken on a daily basis in order to maximize its beneficial effect.

There was also a timing issue. Joe confided that he thought the medication worked better when he took it after a meal rather than before eating. He was definitely eating before bedtime, and told me that he often had a bedtime snack consisting of a few cookies and a glass of milk.

I ordered a barium swallow (a diagnostic procedure described in Chapter 3) to confirm the presence of reflux of acid from the stomach up into the esophagus. This showed that Joe indeed had what we call wide open reflux, a condition in which stomach acid constantly moves upward into the esophagus. No other abnormalities were identified, so no further testing of his esophagus was felt to be necessary.

I explained to Joe that the reason his heartburn wasn't getting better was the fact that he was not taking the medicine correctly. A lifestyle change was required to maximize the effect of the medication. Acid blockers like omeprazole have to be taken a half hour before the meal on an empty stomach, or 30 minutes before breakfast and 30 minutes before the evening meal. He had to avoid snacking at bedtime.

I told Joe not to have anything to eat within two hours of going to bed. He was instructed to raise the head of his bed on blocks so that his head was higher than his feet, allowing a better chance for acid to stay in his stomach rather than flowing up into his esophagus.

Obesity also played a role. Over the years, Joe's increasing belly fat had resulted in stomach acid being pushed up into his esophagus, resulting in heartburn. If he lost some weight, this would definitely help his heartburn.

Over the next six months, Joe became much better at taking his medications as prescribed. I enlisted his wife's assistance in helping Joe stay on schedule when it came to taking his acid blockers. I also asked her to monitor his food intake after supper and especially at bedtime.

Eventually, Joe's heartburn symptoms improved as did his ability to sleep through the night. He was eventually referred to our Obesity Center and was evaluated for bariatric surgery to control his obesity. Stomach surgery to control food intake has proven to be very successful in reducing blood pressure, diabetes, and reflux symptoms in obese patients.

Takeaways

1. Lack of adherence to a medication schedule is one of the major reasons for failure of treatment in patients with reflux.

2. Eating at bedtime, even a few cookies and milk, makes the stomach produce acid at night and leads to nocturnal heartburn.

3. Obesity is the most common cause of heartburn in our society, and is also a major contributor to high blood pressure, diabetes, and cardiovascular disease including heart attacks and strokes.

Evie Brooks' case history: "Will my heartburn go away after the baby arrives?"

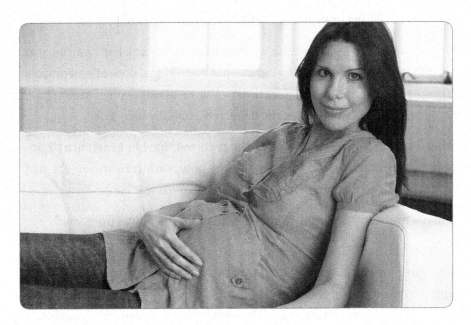

I treated Evie Brooks during the third trimester of her first pregnancy. She reported that approximately a month before her initial consultation with me, she started having severe heartburn and regurgitation of food and fluid into the back of her throat. Her obstetrician told her to take some Tums, a popular antacid tablet. She followed this advice, but the tablets only provided temporary and partial relief.

Evie reported that she had gained 28 pounds during the pregnancy. Prior to pregnancy she had not suffered from heartburn except for an occasional bout after a heavy meal or spicy food. The diagnosis of acid reflux was quite obvious from her story and her situation. As expected, physical examination showed a very pregnant lady whose huge uterus was squeezing her stomach and pushing stomach acid and food up into her esophagus.

I advised Evie to do the following:

1. Start taking the acid-blocking medication omeprazole (Prilosec) at a dose of 20 mg in the morning before breakfast.

2. Elevate the head of her bed.

3. Avoid lying down after a meal.

4. Avoid eating or drinking anything within 2 hours of bedtime.

When I saw her a week later, she was much better, but still had heartburn at night that was really disturbing her sleep. An additional dose of omeprazole 20 mg in the late afternoon before the evening meal was enough to eliminate her heartburn. Six weeks later she delivered a healthy baby girl.

When I saw Evie about a year later, she reported that her heartburn disappeared after delivery and she stopped the omeprazole. However, she had gradually gained 20 pounds, and now the heartburn was back.

"I'm not pregnant," she said. "But I feel like I did when I was pregnant."

I started her back on the omeprazole and suggested that weight loss might help, given the relationship to the heartburn with the first pregnancy, and with the recent weight gain over the past year. Just like pregnancy, additional fat in the abdomen pushes up on the stomach and contributes to reflux of acid. As we learned in the previous case, the same thing can happen in men who develop obesity. Heartburn and reflux often follow.

Weight loss is a difficult goal, despite all of the help patients can get in the form of diets, exercise, appetite suppressants, and when all else fails, bariatric surgery. However, Evie was motivated to lose weight and feel better. She also did not want to continue taking omeprazole indefinitely. She started on a strict weight reduction diet, and over the subsequent eight months she returned to her original pre-pregnancy weight of 135 pounds. At the same time, her heartburn gradually diminished, and she eventually got off the daily omeprazole for good.

Takeaways

Evie's case illustrates several important points:

1. As with obesity, pregnancy can push up on the stomach and contribute to reflux of acid.
2. Weight loss can permanently control heartburn in some patients.
3. Lifestyle changes and medication are both effective at treating mild heartburn.

However, as we will see in the next case, medications don't work for everyone.

Dana Lynch's case history: "Can my acid blocking medications lead to Alzheimer's?"

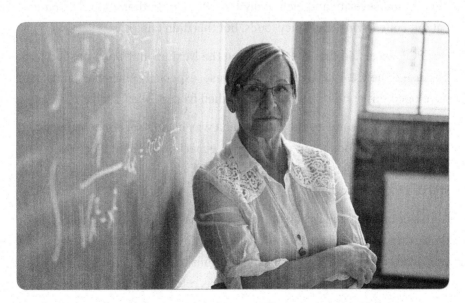

Dana Lynch was a 64-year-old college professor with a history of heartburn which started in her 30s. She was initially treated with H2 blockers (a type of acid blocker for moderate symptoms) on an on-and-off basis. Around age 50, she was started on the medication Nexium, a proton pump inhibitor (PPI) that is used to treat acid reflux. She took 1 tablet per day in the morning before breakfast. She reduced consumption of trigger foods like red wine and coffee, and avoided eating or drinking at bedtime. Dana was fit and active and kept her weight down.

About a year before she first consulted with me, Dana was told by some friends that she should not take Nexium or any PPI medications because they were associated with cognitive decline or Alzheimer's disease. She and her husband discussed this with her primary care physician (PCP), who told them that a few studies had indeed linked proton pump inhibitors with increased cognitive decline as well as other side effects such as reduced calcium absorption and renal failure. The PCP instructed Dana to slowly taper off the Nexium and use antacid tablets like Tums or Rolaids to control heartburn that might occur after she stopped the Nexium.

Three months later, Dana was off the Nexium. She controlled the minimal heartburn with antacid tablets. But the heartburn gradually increased in frequency and severity and eventually became very bothersome. The patient cut out coffee, wine, and spicy foods, but this didn't help.

Her PCP suggested that she go back on the Nexium, but Dana pushed back because of her fear of Alzheimer's disease, especially since her father had developed this condition at age 64 and died from it 3 years later.

By the time she came to the office, Dana was having severe heartburn and regurgitation of food up into her throat, especially at night. She was taking 6 to 8 antacid tablets per day, which helped for a few minutes only. She was still in a lot of discomfort.

At this point, the choices had narrowed down to two options: either go back on Nexium or consider anti-reflux surgery. Given her family history, Dana was firmly opposed to taking any medications that might increase her risk of developing Alzheimer's. Eventually she was referred for anti-reflux surgery.

Takeaways

1. Severe cases of acid reflux require intensive treatment with a special class of medications called acid blockers. There are two types: H2 blockers and proton pump inhibitors (see Chapter 4).

2. Researchers in Germany have identified a potential connection between a type of acid blocker known as a proton pump inhibitor (PPI) and Alzheimer's disease. However, the research is not conclusive (see Chapter 4).

3. Surgical procedures, or anti-reflux operations, are a good alternative to medications for a small number of patients (see Chapter 5).

Jeremy Lee's case history: "What are the surgical alternatives?"

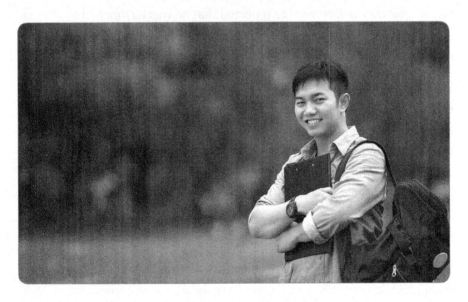

Jeremy Lee was a 19-year-old college freshman at MIT with a career plan to study biomedical engineering or possibly go to medical school. During his first semester at college, Jeremy started experiencing heartburn after eating. This gradually worsened to the point where he was avoiding food and had dropped a few pounds in weight. He went to the student health service and received a diagnosis of probable heartburn that was treated with antacid pills and a recommendation to avoid alcohol, coffee, and spicy food.

He improved briefly, but after a week or so on the antacids and a shift in diet, the heartburn symptoms returned and became much more severe than they were before. Jeremy was experiencing discomfort frequently during the day, but especially at night. He would awaken with severe burning pain in his esophagus and regurgitation of food in the back of his throat. He was having trouble studying and making classes, and had to give up his spot on the college tennis team.

Jeremy was eventually referred for gastrointestinal evaluation and underwent an upper endoscopy that showed bad reflux esophagitis. He was started on omeprazole twice per day and was advised to avoid all food and drinks within two hours of bedtime. As before, Jeremy responded briefly to the acid blocker but eventually reported that he was having bad heartburn around the clock despite excellent adherence to his recommended medications and lifestyle measures.

When I interviewed Jeremy in the office for the first time, it was clear that he was interested in exploring other treatment options for reflux. He told me he could not imagine taking daily medication for the rest of his life unless there were no other options. I presented Jeremy with some information about surgery for reflux and also mentioned the recently approved LINX prosthesis. He was very interested in this novel approach, that was now available at our hospital as an option for those patients seeking surgical relief of reflux symptoms.

During his next summer break, Jeremy was admitted to our surgical department and had the LINX device placed around his lower esophagus. He was discharged home on the day after surgery. During the first few weeks after the procedure, Jeremy had some difficulty swallowing, but eventually this disappeared. When I saw him a few months after the operation, Jeremy was symptom-free and working as a tennis instructor at a summer camp in New Engand.

Takeaways

Jeremy's case demonstrates that even young, previously healthy people can experience acid reflux. Nearly one in ten patients with reflux-related diagnoses are 34 or younger (see Figure 3).

Figure 3: Age of patients with reflux-related diagnoses

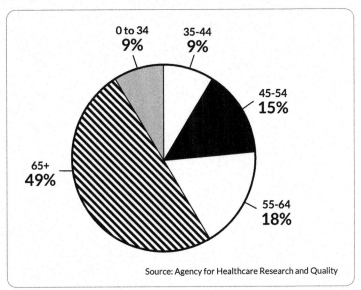

Source: Agency for Healthcare Research and Quality

Other takeaways include:

1. A special procedure called an upper endoscopy (see Chapter 3) can help doctors diagnose severe cases of acid reflux.

2. Acid blockers and lifestyle changes may be ineffective in some patients.

3. Surgical procedures can offer relief for patients who fail to respond to medication, but they are typically seen as last resorts.

The LINX prosthesis and other surgical procedures for the treatment of acid reflux are described in more detail in Chapter 5.

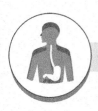

CHAPTER 2

Why heartburn and acid reflux occur

Figure 4: The human stomach

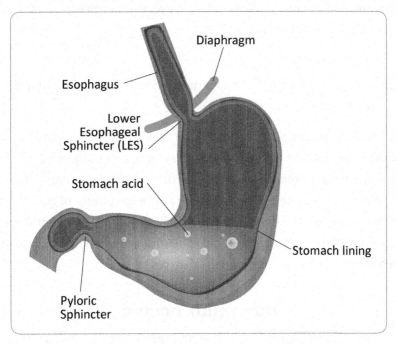

Most people don't think too much about their stomachs. But understanding what this organ does every time you eat a meal is the key to understanding heartburn and acid reflux.

How your stomach works

Think of the stomach as a grinder or mixer. After you swallow food, it travels down your esophagus and then enters the stomach, whose main function is to grind up food and mix it with stomach acid and digestive enzymes.

Acid is normally prevented from flowing upwards into the esophagus by a small but very important muscular valve called the *lower esophageal sphincter (LES)* located at the bottom of the esophagus, just where it joins the stomach as it passes through the diaphragm (see Figure 4). This valve opens automatically when we swallow food and closes after the food passes into the stomach.

Specialized cells in the lining of the stomach secrete about one quart (approximately one liter) of stomach acid every time you eat. Stomach acid has two important functions:

1. Digesting food
2. Killing harmful viruses and germs that sometimes are found in food and water.

Sphincters, which are small muscles that act as valves to control the flow between different parts of your digestive system, determine what happens next. After we eat, stomach acid mixed with food and liquid normally flows downward through the *pyloric sphincter* at the lower end of the stomach into the *duodenum,* the first part of the small intestine. Soon after it enters the duodenum, the hydrochloric acid is neutralized by sodium bicarbonate secreted from the gallbladder and the pancreas.

How reflux occurs

After a meal, the stomach is filled with food and drink, plus gastric juice secreted by the stomach. The stomach has an impressive capacity to hold a lot of food and drink, which it slowly grinds up and releases into the small intestine where most of the nutrients are absorbed.

Normally, the stomach contents do not flow upwards into the esophagus. That's because when we are not eating, the lower esophageal sphincter—the valve at the lower end of the esophagus—is closed tightly to keep stomach acid where it belongs: in the stomach.

But if the LES is weak and doesn't close completely, then acid and food will travel upward into the esophagus (see Figure 5).

Figure 5: Sphincters in open and closed states

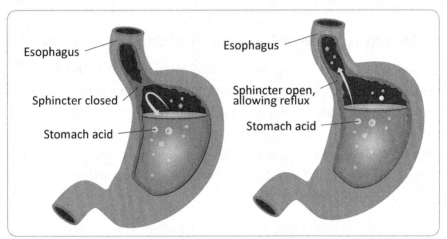

The lining of the esophagus is very sensitive to the burning effect of acid. *Heartburn* is the term we use to describe the discomfort experienced when stomach acid *refluxes* (moves back up) into the esophagus. Nearly everyone experiences a bout of heartburn once in a while, especially after a rich meal.

If this reflux occurs and the patient suffers from heartburn symptoms daily, or more than three times per week for a period of 6 weeks, then we diagnose acid reflux. The medical term for this condition is known as *GERD* or *gastro-esophageal reflux disease.*

What the research says: For primary care physicians, about 1 in 20 patient consultations are related to GERD. (Source: *Journal of the American Board of Family Medicine,* 2005.)

Some reflux patients report regurgitation of food into the throat and mouth. When someone states, "I can't eat barbeque or chili because they always repeat on me," they are describing the taste of food that is being regurgitated or refluxed up the esophagus into the throat and then re-swallowed.

Another way to think about the gastrointestinal (GI) tract is to compare it to a one-way street. What goes in the mouth is intended to flow through the system in one direction only—that is, downwards. Anything that backs up the system is likely to cause problems, just like two-way traffic on a one-way street.

Heartburn symptoms: variations on a theme

Doctors and researchers are not sure why the sphincter valve above the stomach is weak in patients with reflux. The condition can start anytime, from infancy to old age. It's not related to an infection or irritation, and often occurs in people who are otherwise fit and healthy. Patients describe the uncomfortable sensation of acid in the esophagus as "heartburn," because the discomfort is felt behind the breastbone at the lower end of the chest, right in front of the heart.

Like most medical conditions, heartburn can produce a variety of symptoms, and can be described in many different ways. Sometimes, reflux pain radiates up into the neck or straight through to the back between the shoulder blades. Bad heartburn can be so acute and severe that patients and their doctors may think they are having a *myocardial infarction* (MI), commonly known as a heart attack.

Other symptoms of reflux include:

> ➤ A sour or acid sensation in the back of the throat.

> ➤ The taste of previously swallowed food in the back of the throat.

> ➤ Regurgitation of stomach fluid or food up into the throat.

> ➤ Coughing, especially at night or when lying down.

> ➤ Constant throat clearing or changes in the voice.

In patients with severe, long-standing reflux, acid can irritate the *larynx* (voice box) and lungs and cause hoarseness, wheezing, cough, and even pneumonia.

A small fraction of patients feel nauseated or queasy when acid refluxes into the esophagus. This sensation typically occurs in the morning when the stomach is empty. In women of childbearing age, morning nausea can be confused with pregnancy, itself a major trigger of heartburn.

Some other factors can also increase the risk of heartburn and GERD. Regular use of certain drugs (see list, below), especially aspirin and pain relievers such as ibuprofen and naproxen, can lead to irritation and inflammation of the esophagus. Medicines used to treat *osteoporosis* or bone loss can irritate the esophagus, so patients taking medications such as Fosamax are advised to stay upright for at least 30 minutes after taking these kinds of meds to ensure complete emptying of the esophagus.

Drugs that increase the risk of acid reflux	
Pain relievers	**Osteoporosis medications**
Aspirin	Alendronate (Fosamax)
Ibuprofen	Etidronate (Didronel)
Naproxen	Ibandronate (Boniva)
Motrin	Pamidronate (Aredia)
Aleve	Risedronate (Actonel, Atelvia) Tiludronate (Skelid)

Sources: Author, NIH.gov

Patients who are confined to bed for a long time after a major operation or injury may develop reflux. Lying flat in bed favors reflux because gravity no longer helps to keep acid moving downward. An additional anatomic factor in acid reflux is the presence of a *hiatus hernia* (also called *hiatal hernia*), a fairly common condition in which the stomach pushes upward through the diaphragm into the chest. Many patients with reflux have a hiatus hernia, and this is more common with age. (A *hernia* is a general term that means an organ has moved from its usual location into another space or region of the body.) Although a hiatus hernia is seldom by itself a cause of reflux, it is often identified in patients who come to the doctor because of heartburn.

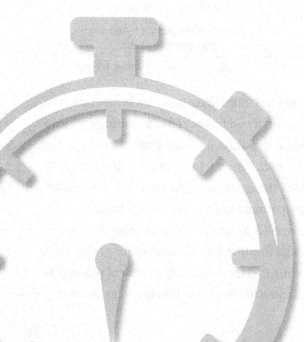

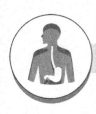

CHAPTER 3

Diagnosis of acid reflux and GERD

Your doctor can usually diagnose acid reflux on the basis of your symptoms. In fact, most patients with reflux know what's wrong even before they visit their doctor. In patients with these typical symptoms, tests like endoscopy or X-ray tests are usually not required to make the diagnosis of reflux.

However, other conditions of the stomach and esophagus can cause similar symptoms. If the diagnosis isn't clear-cut, then diagnostic tests may be needed to identify other problems:

➤ Gallstones can sometimes cause squeezing or burning pain in the chest after eating.

➤ Heart pain, also called *angina*, occurs in the lower chest and sometimes is worse at night.

➤ Stomach inflammation (*gastritis*) and ulcers can easily be confused with acid reflux symptoms, and also respond to acid blockers and antacids.

A careful medical history is sufficient by itself to make a diagnosis in 80% to 90% of cases of acid reflux. It's the other 10% to 20% that require more tests to rule out other conditions whose symptoms overlap with reflux.

Sometimes your doctor may be unable to tell for sure if your symptoms are related to reflux or to some other condition. For instance, patients may experience typical reflux symptoms, but the acid-blockers don't seem to work. These cases are often sent to a *gastroenterologist*, also known as a GI doctor. These specialists concentrate on diseases of the digestive system, and may be able to clarify the situation and recommend treatments. The GI doctor may order some of the tests described here to sort out the problem and help improve the treatment plan.

Barium swallow

One of the first and simplest tests we order for diagnosing reflux is a *barium swallow* or *upper GI series* in which the patient swallows a few cups of barium. The white, chalky liquid shows up on an X-ray of the esophagus and stomach (see image, below).

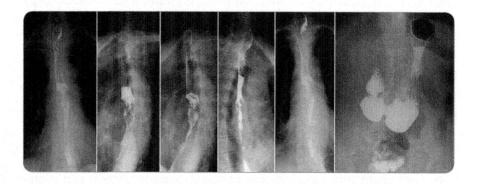

What we look for is reflux of the barium in the stomach back up into the esophagus. The radiologist will ask the patient to lie down on the X-ray table after swallowing the barium to maximize the flow of barium back up into the esophagus. This is a simple and non-painful test, and does not expose the patient to very much radiation.

Typically, this test is positive in patients with mild-to-moderate reflux. In some patients with severe reflux, barium may travel from the stomach all the way up the esophagus and into the throat.

A barium swallow test can also diagnose a *hiatus hernia*, a frequent finding in patients with heartburn and GERD. In patients with a hiatus hernia, the top part of the stomach slides upward through the diaphragm into the chest. This condition, also known as *hiatal hernia,* is caused by weakness of the diaphragm that allows the top of the stomach to migrate into the chest (see Figure 6).

Figure 6: Hiatal hernia

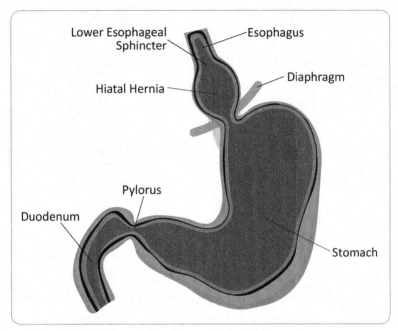

Patients sometimes become concerned when they hear that their barium swallow shows a hiatus hernia, because they think they may need to have it fixed surgically, as is usually the case with an inguinal or groin hernia.

However, we don't often recommend surgery for a hiatus hernia unless we are going to recommend an operation to reduce reflux.

Upper endoscopy

In patients with more advanced or complicated reflux, the GI doctor may recommend *upper endoscopy*. The endoscope is a flexible tube about the width of your little finger with a light on the end that is passed through the mouth into the throat (see Figure 7). This tool lets doctors directly examine the lining on the inside of the esophagus, stomach, and upper small intestine.

Figure 7: Upper endoscopy

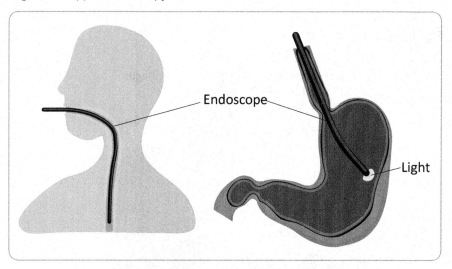

Serious cases of acid reflux can irritate the lining of the esophagus, and cause redness, swelling, irritation, and even small ulcerations that can bleed and cause pain. In some patients, endoscopy can let the GI specialist identify other causes of symptoms like nausea or pain, including inflammation or infection of the stomach, or stomach ulcers that can mimic reflux symptoms.

Bravo 48-hour pH probe

The most accurate test for heartburn is a 48-hour acid reflux study which measures the frequency and intensity of acid reflux from the stomach into the esophagus. This test requires endoscopy to attach a miniature pH detector the size of a large vitamin pill to the bottom of the esophagus (see Figure 8). Attaching the probe is not painful, and the patient cannot feel that the probe is there.

Figure 8: Bravo capsule and receiver

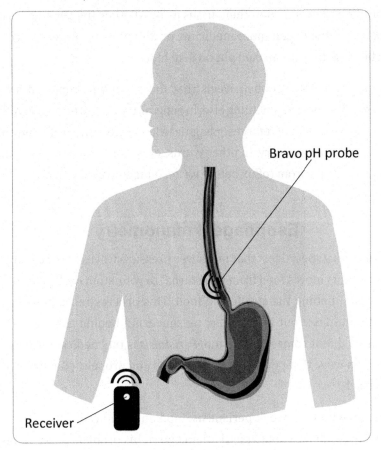

The patient goes home with the probe in place, and can eat and drink normally. The acid level is wirelessly transmitted for the next 48 hours to a recorder the size of a deck of cards that patients wear on their belts or clothing. When they feel heartburn or other symptoms, they press an event button on the recorder. Later, when the probe results are interpreted, the pain event can be correlated with the acid level (or pH level) recorded simultaneously by the probe in the esophagus.

The Bravo 48-hour pH recording is the gold standard for the diagnosis of acid reflux, and helps a GI doctor decide on the type of medical or surgical therapy. For example, about 40% of patients with a diagnosis of reflux are still not much better after they are treated with lifestyle changes and acid-blockers. The question then arises as to whether the treatment is not adequate and they need more medicine, or if they need surgery to correct reflux because they are maxed out on acid blockers.

Sometimes the Bravo probe reveals that the symptoms reported are not related to reflux but to something else. In general, patients who are candidates for surgical treatment of reflux esophagitis will require a Bravo pH study prior to consideration of surgery. In other words, we want to be really sure that a patient is suffering from reflux before we recommend an operation.

Esophageal manometry

Manometry is a special test that measures pressure waves in the esophagus. The esophagus moves food from your throat to your stomach by contracting (or pushing) behind the swallowed food. This process resembles the way you get toothpaste out of the tube, by squeezing behind the paste inside the tube so that it comes out the top. *Peristalsis* is the medical term for this contraction wave that pushes behind the food and propels it downward into the stomach.

In patients who have weak peristalsis, food and fluid can take a long time to travel through the esophagus. Patients with this problem make complain of food sticking in the esophagus and may also have heartburn. Manometry may be combined with a 48-hour pH test mentioned above to give a complete picture of the function of the esophagus.

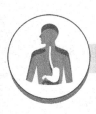

CHAPTER 4

Basic treatment of acid reflux

Acid reflux is one of the most common conditions encountered in medical practice. Most people have at least one or two episodes of heartburn per year, especially after a large or spicy meal, or drinking too much alcohol, coffee, or acidic juice.

Occasional heartburn should not raise any alarms, and does not require a visit to your doctor or GI specialist. However, when heartburn is persistent for more than a month or two, or does not respond to simple measures like dietary changes or antacid tablets like Tums or Rolaids, then a visit to your physician is a good idea.

Antacids	
Alka-Seltzer	Riopan
Maalox	Tums
Mylanta	Gaviscon
Rolaids	

Source: American Gastroenterological Association

One of the most important reasons to get checked by a doctor is because heartburn can be mistaken for other causes of chest discomfort, including the following ailments:

➤ *Angina pectoris*, which indicates a problem with blood flow to the heart muscle.

31

➤ Gallstones, which can sometimes cause pain in the chest or right side of the abdomen.

➤ Lung conditions such as pleurisy, pneumonia, or a *pulmonary embolism* (blood clot).

Treatment of reflux disease depends on the severity and frequency of the symptoms. In patients with at least two episodes of heartburn per week, we typically recommend lifestyle modifications, and a medication to block acid production from the stomach.

Lifestyle modifications refer to simple measures that can help limit or even eliminate heartburn:

➤ We recommend weight loss for patients who have had recent weight gain or who have always been overweight or obese but have recently developed heartburn.

➤ We often recommend that the patient seek out help from a nutritionist for dietary advice or possibly discuss with their primary care doctor a medication to help reduce appetite.

➤ Reduction of 10% of body weight can sometimes reduce the symptoms of reflux. As a bonus, weight loss is also a good way to reduce the risk of heart attacks, strokes, and diabetes.

Another lifestyle measure is raising the head of the bed 6 to 8 inches (15 to 20 centimeters). Gravity can help the esophagus empty during sleep, when acid typically runs up into the esophagus in patients suffering from heartburn. The idea is to place the head and shoulders higher than the stomach and hips, to allow drainage of acid from the esophagus into the stomach. There are a few ways to do this:

➤ A simple approach is to place blocks of thick wood or heavy books under the legs or bed frame at the head of the bed.

➤ Another useful maneuver is a foam wedge pillow which elevates the top part of the body.

➤ We recommend that patients do not use extra standard pillows, because this may cause a bend in the abdomen which can actually increase heartburn.

The overall idea is to keep the body flat in bed but with the head higher than the hips.

Trigger foods

A very important lifestyle recommendation for reflux patients is to avoid *trigger foods* that they have identified as a cause of heartburn. On this list of no-no's are many of the daily pleasures of life:

➤ Coffee

➤ Chocolate

➤ Alcohol

➤ Acidic or rich foods like meat sauces, spaghetti sauce, oranges and grapefruits

➤ Foods containing wine or other acidic components.

Other risky foods and drinks are included in the list below.

Trigger foods	
Fried or fatty foods	Wine
Chocolate	Alcoholic drinks
Peppermint	Coffee
Mustard	Carbonated drinks
Vinegar	Fruit juice
Ketchup and tomato sauce	Citrus fruits

Source: American Gastroenterological Association

Going to bed or napping with a full stomach is not a good idea for patients who are experiencing heartburn or reflux. Therefore, avoid eating within two hours before bedtime or before lying down for a nap. Very tight clothing can increase the risk of heartburn by increasing pressure in the abdomen, so loose fitting, comfortable clothing is recommended.

Cessation of cigarette smoking is recommended to all patients, as smoking irritates the esophagus and increases the severity of heartburn.

Acid-blocking medications

Acid blockers that reduce the production of stomach acid are the mainstay of our medical treatment for acid reflux. There are two major types of acid blockers: *Histamine blockers (H2 blockers)* and *proton pump inhibitors (PPIs)*.

H2 blockers

The histamine blockers, such as cimetidine, ranitidine, and their relatives were introduced in the late 1970s. Cimetidine, also known by the brand name Tagamet, came on the market in 1977, and was one of the first GI blockbuster drugs to top yearly sales of $1 billion. Generic versions of cimetidine are now available.

Histamine blockers revolutionized the treatment of ulcer disease and heartburn. Prior to cimetidine, we had no drugs to block stomach acid, and had to rely on antacid tablets and so-called "ulcer diets" of bland foods and cream. Such diets were not very effective (and for some patients, were not very healthy, either).

Histamine blockers have been used for decades and are considered very safe and effective. These medications are now available over the counter, and can also be prescribed by your doctor if higher drug dosing or permanent use is necessary.

H2 blockers
Famotidine (Pepcid AC, Pepcid Oral)
Cimetidine (Tagamet, Tagamet HB)
Ranitidine (Zantac, Zantac 75, Zantac)
Efferdose, Zantac injection, and Zantac Syrup)
Nizatidine Capsules (Axid AR, Axid Capsules)

Source: medlineplus.gov

If you have bothersome heartburn that requires long-term medication for more than a month, then you should discuss these medications with your doctor. Histamine H2 blockers are considered excellent treatment for mild-to-moderate heartburn, without complications.

Proton pump inhibitors (PPIs)

In patients with more advanced or severe reflux, we generally recommend a proton pump inhibitor such as omeprazole or lansoprazole (see list, below). There are now various proton pump inhibitor (PPI) medications on the market, all very similar in their modes of action and effectiveness. They are available over the counter and also by prescription.

Your health insurance will probably only cover one or two of these medications, and sometimes in only a low dose or for a limited time. Your doctor can prescribe one that your insurance covers, since the co-pay will generally be cheaper than buying it yourself over the counter.

PPIs are the most powerful inhibitors of stomach acid currently available for treatment of reflux. If you need these medications for long-term use (six weeks or more) you should be under the care of your primary care doctor or gastroenterologist who can supervise the use of these medications and advise you about what benefits and side effects to expect.

Proton Pump Inhibitors
Omeprazole (Prilosec)
Esomeprazole (Nexium)
Lansoprazole (Prevacid)
Rabeprazole (AcipHex)
Pantoprazole (Protonix)
Dexlansoprazole (Dexilant)

Source: medlineplus.gov

We generally reserve the use of proton pump inhibitors like omeprazole for patients who have not improved sufficiently with lifestyle changes and use of H2 blockers. PPIs are taken on a daily basis, usually in the morning, 30 minutes before breakfast. Sometimes we recommend an 8-week course of omeprazole to treat heartburn and then see if we can discontinue the medication. Eight weeks is usually sufficient to heal esophagitis and improve or eliminate heartburn.

We consider all the medications shown in the list above to be equivalent, although some patients may respond better to one rather than another. Some doctors may recommend one brand based on their experience with a particular drug, but their potency and side effects are about the same.

What the research says: In 2004, there were an estimated 64.6 million prescriptions for gastroesophageal reflux disease (GERD), compared to 2 million for hemorrhoids. (Source: *The Burden of Digestive Diseases in the United States, 2008.*)

Dealing with PPIs and "acid rebound"

When patients abruptly stop their PPIs instead of tapering off gradually, they may get rebound hyperacidity and severe heartburn. Patients who have taken a PPI for a long time often notice that when they miss even a single dose, they get bad heartburn later in the day. Discontinuation of proton pump inhibitors can be very difficult, even after the heartburn has disappeared for a period of months or even years. Only about 50% of patients are able to stop PPI medications. Heartburn recurs months or years after the initial treatment phase and may require re-treatment, which is usually long-term.

Some patients have symptoms that are relieved partially by lifestyle modifications and treatment, but still have symptoms of reflux, and generally are referred to a gastroenterologist for decisions on therapy. In patients who are still having symptoms after a single dose per day of omeprazole or a similar therapy, we generally recommend twice-a-day therapy, once in the morning before breakfast and again before the evening meal (with a medication such as omeprazole).

Another approach to patients with GERD which doesn't respond to medication is to add an H2 blocker such as ranitidine at bedtime.

Side effects of acid blockers

Acid-blocking drugs have been taken by hundreds of millions of patients worldwide since their discovery in the 1970s. This high usage reflects the huge number of patients with heartburn, gastritis, stomach ulcers, and other GI diseases related to excess stomach acid. These drugs are remarkably effective and have changed how we treat these diseases. Before these drugs were discovered, surgery to treat ulcers and reflux was very common. But nowadays such operations on the stomach are so rarely recommended that most younger surgeons have never even performed one!

But all medications have side effects, and these drugs are no exception. Long-term use of acid blockers is associated with increased risk of infections, particularly intestinal infections and pneumonia. As noted earlier, stomach acid provides a powerful barrier that protects against harmful germs in our food and water. By blocking acid production, we weaken or eliminate this important barrier to infection, allowing more germs to gain entry into our bodies. This is not as bad as it sounds, because our food and water is much cleaner and safer now than it was in earlier times.

Chronic acid blocker therapy causes reduced absorption of magnesium in the intestine, which in turn has been linked to weakened bones and increased risk of hip fractures. Magnesium is a vital mineral necessary for healthy bones. Lower magnesium levels in the blood increases the risk for fractures, especially after age 65. Some patients require supplemental magnesium pills during acid blocker therapy to make sure they don't develop low magnesium levels in the blood and weak bones.

Renal or kidney impairment has also been linked to omeprazole and other proton pump inhibitors. Stopping these drugs usually reverses the kidney failure.

Do acid blockers cause Alzheimer's disease?

One of the most worrisome possible side effects of acid blockers is the relationship to dementia and Alzheimer's disease.

Two recent studies from Germany reported an increased risk of cognitive impairment such as Alzheimer's disease in long-term users of omeprazole and related drugs. However, the studies have been criticized by some doctors and medical societies because of their methods, which involved searching very large databases of patients who carried the diagnosis of dementia, and were also taking or had previously taken a proton pump inhibitor. Such studies do not prove *causation*, but only show an *association*.

We already know that older people are more likely to be prescribed proton pump inhibitors than younger people. Older people are also far more likely to get dementia. Similarly, older people are much more likely than younger people to take a cathartic like prune juice or a stool softener to prevent constipation—but no one has suggested that cathartics could be a possible cause of dementia.

In general, association studies are rather weak compared to randomized double-blinded trials, which would involve putting thousands of healthy patients on either an acid blocker or a placebo (a dummy pill), and following them for five years to compare the incidence of dementia in the two groups. This kind of study is not likely to happen in the near future.

On the other hand, the possibility exists that these German reports may be an early warning sign. When the first association study of a possible causal link between cigarette smoking and lung cancer was published, the American Medical Association and many doctors pushed back and warned against a rush to judgment. But subsequent studies confirmed the link. Eventually this led to a decrease in tobacco use in the United States and then to a significant drop in lung cancer rates.

In recent years, quite a few of my reflux patients have been advised by their doctors or a family member to stop their omeprazole because of the possibility that these drugs increase the risk of dementia. But simply stopping these types of drugs in patients with bad reflux is not as simple as it sounds. Only 20 to 25% of patients who are long-term users of omeprazole or other PPIs can stop them without experiencing a return of bad heartburn.

While other acid blockers such as H2 blockers are available, they are not as effective as PPIs and have their own side effects. For those patients who experience a return of symptoms when PPIs are stopped, they can consider taking a histamine blocker for a long period of time, or learn more about the surgical options (discussed in the next chapter) to control their reflux symptoms.

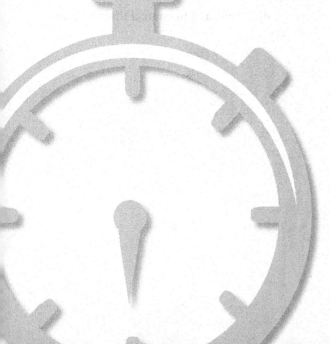

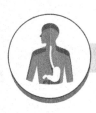

CHAPTER 5

Coping with severe acid reflux

In some patients, acid reflux over months or years can damage the esophagus and lead to complications. Some of the more frequent or typical complications are listed below.

One serious complication of chronic reflux is *stricture formation*, the formation of scar tissue in the esophagus which narrows the opening of the esophagus and causes difficulty in swallowing. Patients complain of food sticking in their throats, especially solid food like meat or apples.

Bad reflux can also cause people to wake up at night with a choking sensation because acid and/or food have passed upward into the throat and entered the airway. This condition, called *aspiration*, can be very frightening to patients who are not aware that they have reflux.

What the research says: Of all people suffering from GERD, 80% report reduced enjoyment of food. (Source: *Journal of the American Board of Family Medicine*, 2005.)

Occasionally, reflux can cause an irritation of the larynx or lung. These patients then complain of cough, hoarseness, frequent throat clearing, or wheezing. Reflux can worsen pre-existing asthma. In some cases, treatment of reflux can lead to less wheezing and easier breathing in asthma patients.

Patients with chronic reflux may also feel a lump in the throat or complain of sore throat, increased dental problems related to acid affecting the teeth, and painful swallowing if there are ulcers in the esophagus.

Barrett's Esophagus and esophageal cancer

About 5% of patients with chronic acid reflux develop a serious precancerous complication called Barrett's Esophagus, an abnormal appearance of the cells lining the esophagus. This can only be diagnosed by endoscopy and biopsy (taking a small tissue sample from the lining of the esophagus).

We recommend endoscopy and biopsy to screen patients for Barrett's esophagus starting 10 years after the onset of GERD. Barrett's Esophagus is a serious but treatable condition, and requires follow-up by a GI doctor with experience and expertise in management of this condition. Barrett's Esophagus is painless, and progresses to cancer of the esophagus in only a very small number of patients.

Acid reflux that doesn't get better: Refractory GERD

About 10% to 25% of patients with reflux esophagitis may complain of persistent symptoms, even after taking the standard doses of acid blockers (such as omeprazole) and following lifestyle recommendations. These patients may feel somewhat better than before treatment, but still notice bothersome heartburn or other symptoms that reduce their quality of life.

Even worse off are those unfortunate patients who come back to the office with little or no improvement despite maximal therapy with medications and excellent adherence to lifestyle changes.

Refractory GERD or heartburn that doesn't respond to the usual medications and lifestyle changes seems to be increasing in frequency in the United States and Europe. Some experts have attributed this to the rising incidence of obesity in many countries.

Figure 9: Obesity rates in the US, UK, and Japan (females)

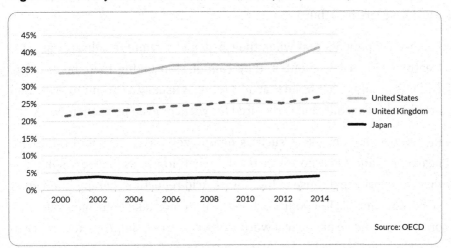

A number of factors besides obesity have been identified in patients with refractory GERD. One big issue is reduced compliance or adherence to the medical regimen or schedule, which happens when patients fail to take acid blocking medications as prescribed. This reduces their effectiveness. I advise my reflux patients that drugs like omeprazole should be taken on an empty stomach 30 minutes before breakfast or dinner. However, about 50% of patients do not follow this plan every day.

There are different patterns of reduced compliance, all of which reduce the effectiveness of the medications:

➤ Taking acid-blocking medications with meals or after eating.

➤ Taking acid blockers at bedtime.

➤ Taking medicine only when they feel heartburn symptoms.

This last pattern is common. Patients may feel some heartburn, and take the medication for a few days and then stop it. When the symptoms recur, as they almost always do, they take the medication again. This on-again, off-again approach is not recommended, as it is far less effective than regular daily use. *Rebound hyperacidity* occurs shortly after stopping an acid blocker, with release of a huge load of acid into the stomach and esophagus, causing severe heartburn.

I advise my patients that when their heartburn symptoms disappear after treatment for a few months, they cannot stop taking their medication. Patients should understand that acid reflux is usually a chronic disease, and acid-blocking medication is required for years or even permanently.

Remember: Acid blockers such as omeprazole or ranitidine do not cure heartburn, and have no effect on the weak lower esophageal sphincter that is the principal cause of heartburn. Acid reduction therapy is aimed at symptom control. Tell your doctor if you cannot take your medication as prescribed, and he or she will work with you to try to improve adherence to a regimen that will help control your symptoms.

What if the acid-blockers don't work?

Failure to respond to acid-controlling medications can sometimes be related to a *hypersensitive esophagus*. Another term for this is *irritable esophagus*, meaning that the lining of the esophagus is very sensitive to even a small amount of acid.

Typically, these patients complain of burning pain in the chest just behind the breast bone, poor response to acid-blocking medications, and there is an absence of any other explanation for the symptoms. Further testing often reveals a normal endoscopy without any evidence of esophageal irritation, and a normal 24-hour pH probe, indicating no evidence for acid reflux.

Patients with hypersensitive esophagus sometimes have significant anxiety or stress in their personal lives that aggravates their heartburn and makes their esophagus overly sensitive. This condition may respond to stress reduction therapy, or may require medications like the tricyclic antidepressant amitriptyline that acts in the brain to reduce the hypersensitivity of the esophagus. Other patients may require stress reduction or anti-anxiety therapy.

Bile reflux

Bile reflux is another cause of refractory GERD. Bile is secreted by the liver and stored in the gallbladder. Bile contains *bile acids* that help digest fat in the diet. After a typical meal, the gallbladder contracts or squeezes, and bile is emptied into the stomach and small intestine. We often find bile in the stomach when we do endoscopy, which is generally not considered to be an abnormality that requires treatment.

But if bile in the stomach is refluxed up into the esophagus, it can be very irritating. It appears that a small number of patients who have refractory GERD may have bile reflux rather than (or in addition to) typical acid reflux. Some of these patients may respond to cholesystramine (Questran), a medicine that binds bile acids, and prevents them from irritating the esophagus. Sometimes we treat bile acid irritation with baclofen, a drug that helps treat heartburn by reducing reflux, not by blocking acid release.

Helicobacter infection

Failure to respond to reflux therapy can be caused by *Helicobacter pylori*, a bacterial infection of the stomach often acquired in childhood. Helicobacter infection leads to inflammation of the lining of the stomach, a condition called *gastritis*.

Some patients have no symptoms of any kind from Helicobacter infection, while others report an upset stomach with pain, fullness and bloating after a meal. These symptoms are called *dyspepsia*, a Greek word that means upset or sore stomach.

The symptoms of Helicobacter infection can sometimes be confused with the symptoms of acid reflux. Acid blockers can help the symptoms of Helicobacter infection, but they don't get rid of the infection. This infection can be eradicated only by intensive antibiotic therapy with two different antibiotics twice per day for 10 days to two weeks. In some parts of the world with poor sanitation and limited access to clean water, Helicobacter can infect more than half of the adult population.

Other conditions that interfere with treatment

Poor response to medical therapy is also seen in patients with GERD who have motility disorders like *diffuse esophageal spasm*, in which strong and persistent muscular contractions of the esophagus cause chest pain. Diagnosis of this condition requires an esophageal motility test.

Certain medications can irritate the stomach, especially arthritis medications such as Aleve and nonsteroidal anti-inflammatory drugs (NSAIDs) which are used in high doses to treat patients with arthritis and rheumatism. If possible, patients with GERD should avoid taking anti-inflammatory drugs which can irritate the stomach and the esophagus.

In recent years, we have seen a large number of teenagers or young adults with a new condition called *eosinophilic esophagitis*, which can be associated with heartburn, difficulty swallowing and allergic symptoms such as burning or tingling of the tongue or throat after eating certain foods. Many of these patients have severe heartburn and evidence of acid damage to the esophagus. This diagnosis is made by endoscopy with biopsy of the esophageal mucosa and can be treated both with acid inhibitors and with food elimination diets under the supervision of an allergist.

When medicines fail: Surgery to treat reflux

Anti-reflux surgery is what we recommend when medical therapy fails to provide adequate relief of reflux symptoms. An operation is considered in only 1 or 2 percent of all chronic reflux patients.

The vast majority of patients respond reasonably well to lifestyle measures and daily therapy with acid blockers like omeprazole or ranitidine. But some patients get only partial relief on these medications, or they do reasonably well, but do not want to take daily medication for the rest of their lives. Lifelong medical therapy can be a heavy burden, especially in younger patients who do not take any other medication and are completely healthy except for acid reflux.

The most frequent indication for surgical treatment is *refractory GERD*, or symptoms that persists despite maximal therapy. A typical patient is a middle-aged person with mild obesity and mild hypertension, but is otherwise healthy. Acid-blocker medications may help partially, but the patient is still feeling heartburn, nausea and other symptoms. Often, they are taking maximal doses of omeprazole, 40 mg twice per day, but they are still symptomatic. Patients like this are ready to consider surgery, as medical therapy is simply not working.

Evaluation of patients for anti-reflux surgery

Before sending GERD patients for a surgical consultation, we want to make sure that their symptoms are really related to reflux and not to something else, such as gallstone disease, Helicobacter infection of the stomach, alcohol abuse, gastric ulcers, or severe gastritis.

Another serious condition that can mimic heartburn is gastroparesis, a condition that limits the ability of the stomach after a meal. This is seen most often in diabetics and is called *diabetic gastroparesis*, but it can occur in some patients who are not diabetic (which is called *idiopathic gastroparesis).*

The following are tests often performed prior to anti-reflux surgery:

➤ Upper endoscopy to rule out other conditions that mimic reflux.

➤ Esophageal manometry to confirm the presence of a weak lower esophageal sphincter.

➤ Barium swallow to assess for hiatus hernia or short esophagus.

➤ Gastric emptying study to make sure that the stomach is able to contract normally after a meal and move food into the small intestine.

Surgical treatment of reflux

The most common surgical treatment for reflux esophagitis is a *laparoscopic Nissen fundoplication* (see Figure 10), in which the surgeon wraps the top of the stomach around the bottom of the esophagus, which strengthens the sphincter valve and prevents acid from going up into the esophagus after a meal.

This operation does not require a large incision, but relies on the use of an operating scope inserted into the abdomen through small incisions called *portholes*. The operation takes a few hours to perform, and patients are typically sent home after a brief hospital stay of a day or two.

Figure 10: Nissen fundoplication

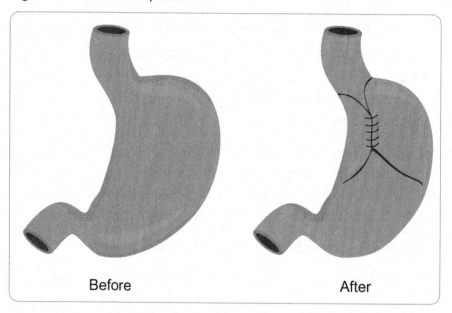

Before   After

This is a highly successful operation: about 90% of patients who have it report long-term improvement in their heartburn symptoms. Some patients still have to take acid blocking medication after the operation, but usually at a lower dosage than before the surgery.

Patients should understand that there are some complications associated with this procedure, both short-term and long-term. As with any operation, infection of the skin incision, a post-operative wound infection, can be expected in up to 5% of patients. These minor infections usually respond quickly to antibiotic therapy.

Some patients pick up a urinary tract infection or intestinal infection during their stay in the hospital. However, these are usually minor and respond to antibiotic therapy.

Longer-term complications of reflux surgery include difficulty swallowing, especially if the surgeon wraps the stomach too tightly around the esophagus. Some patients have persistent or severe postoperative *dysphagia* (difficulty swallowing), and require a second operation to loosen the wrap.

Gassy distention, bloating, and an inability to belch occurs in 10% to 15% of patients after anti-reflux surgery, a complication called *gas bloat syndrome*. This may respond to simethicone pills which break up gas bubbles, or special medications to improve gastric emptying. Re-operation is only rarely required in patients with chronic gas bloat syndrome or difficulty swallowing after the operation.

The LINX device

This recent invention is being increasingly used to treat patients with refractory GERD. The device consists of a ring of magnets, similar to a small bracelet, which is placed around the lower esophagus to keep the esophagus closed and prevent acid from refluxing upward (see Figure 11).

Figure 11: LINX procedure

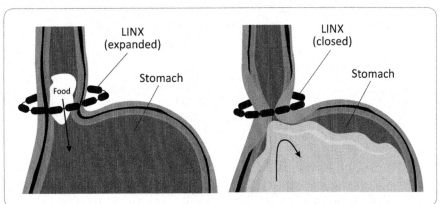

In effect, it is like an artificial sphincter. When the patient swallows, the food travels down the esophagus and overcomes the magnetic force of the bracelet. Then the lower esophagus opens to allow the swallowed food to pass into the stomach. The appeal of the LINX device is that it can be quickly inserted into position, and requires only a short hospital stay for postoperative recovery of a day or so.

Unlike the traditional surgical procedures for acid reflux, patients treated with the LINX device are able to belch or vomit, and seldom develop gas bloat syndrome. In general, this device works as well as traditional surgery, and is likely to become more popular over the next few years.

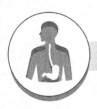

A special request

Thanks for taking the time to read *Acid Reflux & Heartburn In 30 Minutes*. This guide distills the information that I have given to countless patients over the years. I hope it is helpful and reassuring, and can help you better understand available treatments. Of course, any diagnosis and treatment should be made in consultation with your doctor.

I have a special request: **After you have read the book, could you spend a few minutes to review it online? Honest reviews let other readers know what to expect, and also help spread the word that there is hope for people suffering from reflux.** Mentioning the book to your doctor or healthcare provider is another way to raise the profile of *Acid Reflux & Heartburn In 30 Minutes*.

Thanks again for reading the guide.

Dr. J. Thomas Lamont, M.D.

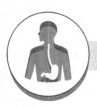

About the author

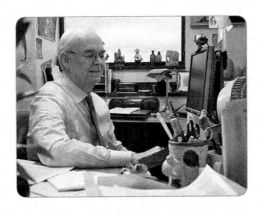

Dr. J. Thomas Lamont received his medical degree in 1965 from the University of Rochester, and was intern, resident, and chief resident in medicine at UCLA.

Following a GI Fellowship at Massachusetts General Hospital, he joined the faculty of Harvard Medical School in 1974. From 1980 to 1995, he was Chief of GI at Boston University School of Medicine, and from 1996 to 2012, was GI Division Chief at Beth Israel Deaconess Medical Center. He has served as Professor of Medicine at Harvard Medical School since 1996. He currently serves as interim Chief of Gastroenterology at Beth Israel Deaconess Medical Center in Boston.

Dr. Lamont's clinical interests are in the area of intestinal infections, GERD, abdominal pain, disorders of intestinal motility, and irritable bowel syndrome.

In addition to his clinical activities, Dr. Lamont serves as a mentor for young scientists and faculty members, and as a resource for manuscript and grant preparation, as well as career planning.

Dr. J. Thomas Lamont served as Associate Editor for GI and Liver Diseases at the *New England Journal of Medicine* from 2001 to 2017, and is currently Editor-in-Chief for Gastroenterology for *UpToDate in Medicine*. He is also the author of *C. Diff In 30 Minutes*.

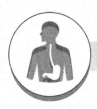

Glossary

Acid blockers – Medications that reduce the production of stomach acid.

Acid reflux – A more serious form of heartburn, also known as GERD.

Agida – Acid indigestion heartburn.

Alzheimer's disease – A progressive brain disorder usually observed in older patients that destroys memory and thinking skills. There is no cure.

Angina pectoris – Indicates a problem with blood flow to the heart muscle.

Antacid tablets – Over-the-counter tablets that can reduce heartburn.

Baclofen – A drug that helps treat heartburn by reducing reflux.

Barium swallow – Also known as an upper GI series, this is a diagnostic procedure in which the patient swallows a few cups of barium, a white chalky liquid that shows up on an X-ray of the esophagus and stomach.

Barrett's Esophagus – An abnormal appearance of the cells lining the esophagus. In a small number of cases, it may progress to esophageal cancer.

Bile – A substance secreted by the liver and stored temporarily in the gallbladder that breaks down fat in your diet

Bile acids – A component of bile designed to help digest fat in the diet.

Bravo 48-hour pH probe – A 48-hour acid reflux study which measures the frequency and intensity of acid reflux from the stomach into the esophagus using a sensor.

Cholesystramine (Questran) – A drug that binds bile acids and prevents them from irritating the esophagus.

Diffuse esophageal spasm – Strong and persistent muscular contractions of the esophagus that cause chest pain.

Digestive enzymes – Helps your body break down and digest your food.

Duodenum – The first part of the small intestine just below the stomach.

Dyspepsia – A Greek word that means upset or sore stomach.

Dysphagia – A medical term used to describe difficulty swallowing.

Esophageal manometry – A test that measures pressure waves in the esophagus, which can confirm the presence of a weak lower esophageal sphincter.

Reflux esophagitis – A condition associated with heartburn, difficulty swallowing, and with allergic symptoms such as burning or tingling of the tongue or throat after eating certain foods. Many of these patients have severe heartburn and evidence of acid damage to the esophagus.

Esophagus – The hollow, muscular tube that connects the throat to the stomach.

Fosamax – A drug used to treat osteoporosis that can also irritate the esophagus.

Gas bloat syndrome – An inability to belch and a feeling of distension or bloating, sometimes associated with anti-reflux surgery.

Gastric juice – A very powerful acid solution produced by the stomach that helps digest our food and kills viruses and germs in food and water.

Gastritis – Inflammation of the lining of the stomach.

Gastroenterologist – Also known as a GI doctor. These specialists concentrate on diseases of the digestive system.

Gastroparesis – A condition that limits the ability of the stomach after a meal. This is seen most often in diabetics and is called diabetic gastroparesis, but can occur in some patients who are not diabetic, so-called idiopathic gastroparesis.

GERD – Gastroesophageal reflux disease. Also known as acid reflux.

Helicobacter pylori – A bacterial infection of the stomach often acquired in childhood that can lead to gastritis, or inflammation of the lining of the stomach.

Hiatus hernia – A condition in which the stomach pushes upward through the diaphragm into the chest.

Histamine blocker (H2 blocker) – A type of acid-blocking medication. Examples include cimetidine and ranitidine. H2 blockers are considered excellent treatment for mild-to-moderate heartburn without complications.

Hydrochloric acid – A corrosive substance which is secreted by your stomach.

Hypersensitive esophagus – Also known as irritable esophagus, a condition in which the lining of the esophagus is very sensitive to even a small amount of acid.

Ibuprofen – Pain reliever that can lead to irritation and inflammation of the esophagus.

Laparoscopic Nissen fundoplication – A procedure in which the surgeon wraps the top of the stomach around the bottom of the esophagus, which strengthens the sphincter valve and prevents acid from going up into the esophagus after a meal.

Larynx – Voice box.

LINX device – A small ring of magnets which is placed around the lower esophagus to keep the esophagus closed and prevent acid from refluxing upward, just like the lower esophageal sphincter is designed to do.

Lower esophageal sphincter (LES) – Sphincter that regulates the flow of food and liquid from the esophagus to the stomach. For most people, the LES prevents stomach acid from flowing upwards into the esophagus.

Myocardial infarction (MI) – A heart attack.

Naproxen – A nonsteroidal anti-inflammatory drug and pain reliever that can cause irritation and inflammation of the esophagus.

Nonsteroidal anti-inflammatory drug (NSAID) – A class of medications including Aleve, ibuprofen and similar medications typically used in high doses to treat patients with arthritis and rheumatism.

Osteoporosis – Bone loss.

Proton pump inhibitor (PPI) – A class of acid-blocking medications used to treat acid reflux. Examples include omeprazole and lansoprazole.

Pyloric sphincter – The muscle regulating the flow of partially digested food and liquid from the stomach to the duodenum, the first part of the small intestine.

Rebound hyperacidity – A condition that sometimes occurs when patients abruptly stop taking proton pump inhibitors (PPIs), instead of tapering off gradually.

Refractory GERD – Bad heartburn that persists despite maximal therapy.

Simethicone pills – Used to break up gas bubbles after anti-reflux surgery.

Sphincters – Small muscles that act as valves to control the flow between different parts of your digestive system.

Stricture formation – The formation of scar tissue in the esophagus which narrows the opening of the esophagus and causes difficulty in swallowing.

Upper endoscopy – A procedure in which an endoscope (a flexible tube with a light on the end) is passed through the mouth into the throat to directly examine the esophagus, stomach, and the top of the small intestine.

Wide open reflux – A condition in which stomach acid constantly moves upward into the esophagus.

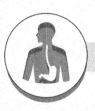

Research & data

The following publications were used as sources of data cited in this book.

"Managing gastroesophageal reflux disease in primary care: the patient perspective." Liker, H., Hungin, P., & Wiklund, I. *Journal of the American Board of Family Medicine*. 2005 Sep-Oct; 18(5): 393-400. https://www.ncbi.nlm.nih.gov/pubmed/16148249

"Statistical Brief #44. Healthcare Cost and Utilization Project (HCUP)." Agency for Healthcare Research and Quality, Rockville, MD. Dec. 2007. http://www.hcup-us.ahrq.gov/reports/statbriefs/sb44.jsp

"Update on the epidemiology of gastro-oesophageal reflux disease: a systematic review." Hashem B El-Serag, Stephen Sweet, Christopher C Winchester, and John Dent. *Gut*. 2014 Jun; 63(6): 871–880. https://www.ncbi.nlm.nih.gov/pmc/articles/PMC4046948/

"OECD.Stat: Health Status." Organization for Economic Cooperation and Development. 2018. http://stats.oecd.org/Index.aspx?DataSetCode=HEALTH_LVNG

"The burden of digestive diseases in the United States." Everhart J.E., editor. US Department of Health and Human Services, Public Health Service, National Institutes of Health, National Institute of Diabetes and Digestive and Kidney Diseases. NIH Publication No. 09-6443, 2008.

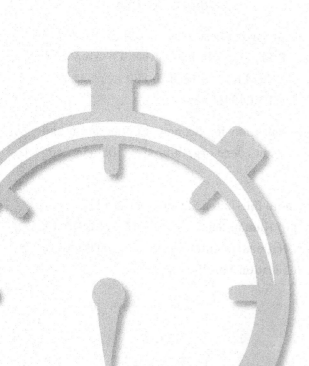

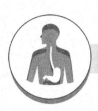

Additional resources

Here are some reliable health information sites for patients interested in learning more about acid reflux and heartburn:

Mayo Clinic (mayoclinic.org): Gastroesophageal reflux disease (GERD)

National Institutes of Health, National Institute of Diabetes and Digestive and Kidney Diseases Health Information Center (www.niddk.nih.gov): Acid Reflux (GER & GERD) in Adults

National Institutes of Health/MedLine Plus (medlineplus.gov): GERD

Note that there are many other web sites and online forums that discuss acid reflux and various treatments. Be very careful about the recommendations and advice published on such sites. While some people have useful experiences to share about dealing with reflux and heartburn, others may be promoting untested, bogus, or even harmful treatments. If you are diagnosed with acid reflux or heartburn, always consult with your doctor about recommended treatment options.

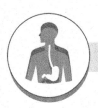

Index

Introduction to
C. Diff In 30 Minutes

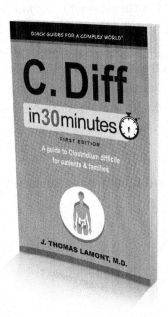

The following bonus chapter is the introduction to C. Diff In 30 Minutes by J. Thomas Lamont, M.D. To download the ebook or purchase the paperback, visit the book's official website, cdiff.in30minutes.com.

Clostridium difficile—commonly referred to as "C. diff"—is a serious bacterial infection of the colon (large bowel). Many people infected with C. diff are sick with diarrhea, abdominal pain, nausea, and weight loss. Others are *carriers* of C. diff, with no signs or symptoms of disease. Some of these carriers have been recently infected with C. diff but have recovered and now feel well. But carriers still have the C. diff organism in their stools and can serve as a silent reservoir of infection in hospitals and nursing homes.

C. diff was first recognized in the 1970s. Since that initial discovery, C. diff has exploded, with more and more cases reported every year in North America, Europe, and further afield. In the past five years, C. diff has spread across the globe, helped in large part by air travel, the availability and frequent use of antibiotics, and the graying of the world's population.

Hospitals in almost every country have reported outbreaks of C. diff. According to a paper published in the *New England Journal of Medicine* in 2015, some 500,000 cases of C. diff are diagnosed in a single year in U.S. hospitals. More than 80% of these cases occurred among Americans aged 65 or older, and approximately 29,000 patients died within 30 days of the initial diagnosis of C. diff. Of 1,000 patients admitted to U.S hospitals, more than 10 will become infected with C. diff. In some hospitals and nursing homes, as many as one in five patients is infected. In recent years, the hospitalization rate for C. diff has increased.

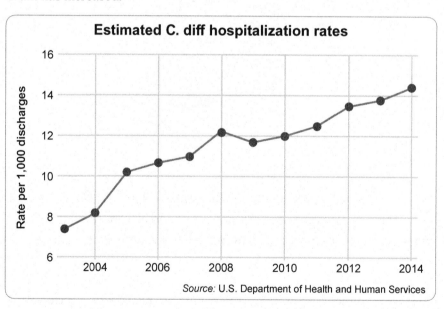

The purpose of this guide is to provide patients and their families with basic information and practical advice about C. diff infection. The number of chronic infections is rising yearly, and many patients (and sometimes their doctors) are not sure what to do next. C. diff is not a simple stomach bug like viral gastroenteritis or food poisoning that disappears in nearly all patients after a week or two. As we discuss in Chapter 3, C. diff can be cured initially by one of these antibiotics:

➤ Metronidazole (sold under the commercial name Flagyl in the United States)

➤ Vancomycin (also called Vanco)

➤ Fidaxomycin (sold as Dificid in the United States)

Unfortunately for many patients, that is not the end of the story. A fundamental problem is the recurrence rate of 15–25%, much higher than we see in any other infection. Some patients suffer multiple recurrences over months or even years. This book is written especially for patients who cannot seem to shake their C. diff, and who get sick with diarrhea again and again.

The situation is not hopeless, though. Even if you have a long-term C. diff infection, you can be helped and eventually cured. The more you understand about your infection, the better you will be able to start on the road to recovery.

If you're interested in learning more about this title, or buying the ebook or paperback, visit the official website located at cdiff.in30minutes.com.